T0144749

Poly-MVA

A New Supplement in the Fight Against Cancer

HOW POLY-MVA AND OTHER PALLADIUM LIPOIC COMPLEXES (LAPds) CAN HELP YOU:

- Improve Overall Health
- Increase Energy & Vitality
- Prevent Cancer
- Heal from Cancer

Robert D. Milne, M.D.,
& Melissa L. Block, M.Ed.

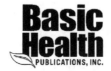

Basic Health PUBLICATIONS, INC.

The information contained in this book is based upon the research and personal and professional experiences of the authors. It is not intended as a substitute for consulting with your physician or other healthcare provider. Any attempt to diagnose and treat an illness should be done under the direction of a healthcare professional.

The publisher does not advocate the use of any particular healthcare protocol but believes the information in this book should be available to the public. The publisher and authors are not responsible for any adverse effects or consequences resulting from the use of the suggestions, preparations, or procedures discussed in this book. Should the reader have any questions concerning the appropriateness of any procedures or preparation mentioned, the authors and the publisher strongly suggest consulting a professional healthcare advisor.

Series Cover Designer: Mike Stromberg
Editor: Carol Rosenberg
Typesetter: Gary A. Rosenberg

Basic Health Guides are published by
Basic Health Publications, Inc.

ISBN: 978-1-59120-049-9 (Pbk.)
ISBN: 978-1-68162-769-4 (Hardcover)

Contents

Introduction

Poly-MVA contains a patented type of palladium lipoic complex—a unique class of nutritional supplements. Palladium lipoic complexes, composed of palladium (a mineral) bonded with lipoic acid (a powerful antioxidant), also contain vitamins, minerals, and amino acids.

Poly-MVA has been found to be a useful nutritional supplement; its ingredients have salutary effects in healthy people, promoting energy production and offering potent antioxidant protection at the cellular level. When used appropriately, Poly-MVA also appears to have the unique capacity to negatively affect anaerobic cells (cells that function without oxygen) while supporting healthy tissues. In fact, Poly-MVA enhances and supports the health of the body while it is fighting cancer—unlike today's arsenal of chemotherapeutic drugs, which often do as much damage as they do good.

Although the research on Poly-MVA is building at present, other palladium lipoic complexes like DNA synthetic reductase are being studied by university scientists. One such compound will soon undergo the U.S. Federal Drug Administration (FDA) approval process. Specific research with Poly-MVA is underway. The purpose of this book is to introduce you to this unique substance and to its remarkable potential. It offers the currently available information so that you can make an educated decision as to why Poly-MVA would be useful to you. Waiting for the results of FDA approval could take years—years that some cancer and chronically ill patients just don't have.

We will primarily emphasize the cancer-fighting benefits of palladium lipoic complexes, because most of the research that has been done has had to do with cancer treatment. Cancer patients are faced with so many frightening choices, and they need thorough explanations of how Poly-MVA may help. The substance's effects on cancer growth are quite amazing, providing results unlike any other compound or nutrient combination. We will, however, also address how Poly-MVA supports health in many other ways.

As research and anecdotal reports accumulate, there is increasing evidence that using Poly-MVA in varying doses for health maintenance may help to prevent cancer and support the body in other ways. Periodically check in with the listings in the Resources section to stay up to date on new information about Poly-MVA and palladium lipoic complexes.

1. A New Paradigm for Healing Cancer

On December 23, 1971, President Richard Nixon signed legislation that officially declared war on cancer. Cancer as a health problem was already growing at a threatening rate, but at the time most people believed that if enough money and scientific effort were thrown at it, cancer could be defeated. With the advent of antibiotic therapy and vaccines, we had defeated so many diseases that had once killed hundreds of thousands of people each year; cancer, it would seem, was just the next foe in line to be decimated by the brilliant minds and advanced technology of the medical research community.

Since then, more than 12 million Americans have died from cancer—approximately 1,500 people each day. That's 45,000 each month. The number of cancer diagnoses continues to rise steadily, as it has throughout the past half century. Cancer is the second leading cause of death in this country. Despite enormous government energy and funding—upward of $45 billion since the war on cancer began—cancer is likely to become the leading cause of death, pushing out cardiovascular disease, by 2012.

Cancer is a far more formidable foe than the Nixon administration realized. It can occur in any one of nearly 100 different forms. Each form can require a different approach to treatment. Even when one therapy works, cancer has a habit of returning in a new and more virulent form. This is why cancer survivors tend to remain vigilant, watching for the return of the disease—particularly within the first five years after remission has been achieved (five years being the threshold at which the individual is thought to be cured).

THE NEWS ISN'T ALL BAD

Success stories are trickling back from the front lines. Through early detection, education, and awareness, oncologists (cancer doctors) can now identify and treat some cancers early enough to greatly improve chances of long-term survival. Although children under the age of fourteen have a higher risk of dying from cancer than any other cause at this point in history, childhood cancer treatments have released many young people from what would once have been a certain death sentence.

The American Association for the Advancement of Science (AAAS) estimates that in 2001 about 8.5 million Americans called themselves cancer survivors. All in all, however, cancer is still a formidable adversary, and it will more than likely continue to grow, affecting more and more people.

The limited progress we've made against cancer with mainstream medical and scientific advances is due to the use of early detection and surgeries, targeted radiation therapies, and chemotherapeutic drugs. These treatments have been the focus of cancer research since the war on cancer began, and improvements on the delivery of these treatments have reduced the damage they inflict on the immune system. This overwhelming emphasis on the treatment of cancer with mainstream medical practices has, however, diverted attention from the primary solution: prevention with integrative (or complementary and alternative) medical approaches.

PREVENTION IS KEY

Many experts agree that many, if not most, forms of cancer are preventable. Some people are more vulnerable to cancer than others because of biological predispositions or genetic factors, but there is much that can be done to prevent cancer within those parameters. The drastic increases in cancer rates over the past century are not due to thunderbolts flung from the heavens. They are more likely due to poor diet, industrial pollutants, smoking, excessive exposure to ultraviolet and other types of radiation, toxic chemicals used to make plastics and other modern materials, pesticides, and a host of other substances that simply did not exist 100 years ago but have become ubiquitous today. Unremitting stress and lack of exercise are also believed to alter the body's chemistry in ways that predispose us to cancer.

Cancer prevention entails doing what one can to avoid chemicals and poisons known to contribute to or cause cancer, and reinforcing the body's natural defenses against cancer with the best possible combination of diet, exercise, and supplements—always keeping in mind that carcinogenesis and cancer promotion are always a combination of nature (genetic and biological factors) and nurture (environmental factors).

In many cases, cancer prevention just isn't an option. The disease has already taken hold in millions of people. Many individuals have genetic or biological predispositions to cancer that have little to do with their lifestyle choices. We need treatments that work and that don't cause side effects that are worse than the disease. We need treatments that don't take such an enormous toll on the body—treatments that work with the body's natural healing energies and processes, without harming the immune and lymphatic systems (two of the body's most important natural defenses against cancer). And we need these treatments right now.

CHANGING THE WAY WE LOOK AT CANCER THERAPY

As you'll learn in the next chapter, cancer is a disruption in the way cells work that causes them to multiply out of control. In the words of Frank Antonawich, Ph.D., one of the scientists who researches the palladium lipoic complexes (one of which is Poly-MVA), cancer is "an invasive event that leads to massive physiological disruption." (F. Antonawich, personal communication with M. Block, October 8, 2003.)

Current cancer therapies focus on the use of highly toxic therapies to try to kill off as many cancerous cells as possible. The collateral damage seen with this approach is considerable. Chemotherapy, radiation, and surgery are notoriously dangerous and can cause severe debility and even death. Because so many cancer patients who undergo these treatments end up dying, it is impossible to know how many of their deaths were at least partly due to these toxic treatment regimens. Sometimes, frankly speaking, the treatments are worse than the disease.

Current therapies typically require that we cut, burn, medicate, and otherwise damage our bodies both physically and mentally in order to rid ourselves of the cancer. The key to winning the war on cancer is to fight it intelligently, with the best tools available.

The ideal treatment for cancer would selectively target cancerous cells, while simultaneously protecting and strengthening healthy cells. Poly-MVA—the new, innovative palladium-lipoic complex—may just achieve this end.

Before we get into the details of how Poly-MVA works, let's establish a basic understanding of what cancer is and how it develops.

2. What Is Cancer?

The cells that make up each of our organs are specialized in their structure and function. Heart cells are designed to contract and release again and again to pump blood. Liver cells are made to filter and neutralize toxins. Lung cells, uterine cells, testicular cells, prostate cells, bone cells, and breast cells are other illustrations of cellular differentiation (specialization).

When the DNA (genetic material) of a healthy, differentiated cell is altered in a way that transforms it into a cancerous cell, the expression of the genes of that cell is changed. This process is known as cancer initiation. The descendants of that cell lose their specialized structure and function, and no longer perform their duties in the body. These cells do not mature into norman cells and are called "undifferentiated."

Genes carry the master instructions to the trillions of cells to function properly. One of the duties of genetic material is to modulate or adjust the growth and death of cells. Proto-oncogenes are genes that, when mutated or otherwise altered, become transformed into oncogenes, genes that promote cancer formation and growth. These proto-oncogenes are strongly affected by environmental influences, such as diet, ultraviolet light, radiation, and smoking. Once these oncogenes have formed, they no longer respond to normal physiological cues, and the stage is set for the development of cancer.

The genetic programming of cancer cells enables them to live as long as they have access to nutrients and a place to grow. Healthy cells are programmed to die after a certain span of time—a form of programmed cell death known as apoptosis. This makes room for new cells to take the place of old ones. In cancerous cells, apoptosis is shut off, and so they grow and multiply unabated, crowding out healthy cells.

CANCER INITIATION—HOW CANCER STARTS

Science's understanding of cancer initiation is constantly improving. Two major categories of initiators have been discovered: toxic chemicals and free radicals.

Toxic Chemicals

Certain chemicals have been found to directly alter cellular DNA in ways that transform healthy cells into cancerous ones. Such chemicals may be synthetic—for example, petroleum products, dioxins, phthalates, and the synthetic estrogens that have been used for hormone replacement therapy—or may be natural, such as the molds that grow on peanuts or certain metals found in nature, such as nickel, arsenic, cadmium, and certain forms of chromium. Even hormones naturally made within the body, such as estrogens, can be carcinogenic if not properly balanced with other hormones.

Free Radicals

Molecules are the basic building blocks of cells, and atoms are the building blocks of molecules. Atoms are made up of a core of protons (which have a positive charge) and neutrons (which have a neutral charge). Electrons (which have a negative charge) orbit around this core. The number of protons, neutrons, and electrons in the atom tell us what element that atom is; atoms are arranged along the periodic table of elements according to these numbers.

A molecule is a group of atoms bonded together in a specific configuration; for example, a water molecule is made up of two hydrogen atoms and one oxygen atom, and a glucose molecule is made up of six carbon atoms, twelve hydrogen atoms, and six oxygen atoms. The bonds between the atoms in a molecule are created by the sharing of a pair of electrons. Electrons, like people, prefer to travel in pairs. When a molecule is split—as it is during the process of metabolism—the electron pairing that held the two now-separated atoms together is also split, and this creates a free radical: a compound that contains an unpaired electron.

Free radicals are highly reactive. Their reactive tendency is to find another electron to form a pair. In the process of acquiring another electron, free radicals react with many kinds of molecules in the body, causing damage to cells and the genetic information they contain. This kind of damage can transform healthy cells into cancerous ones by altering their DNA.

Free radicals will steal electrons from proteins and fats in order to become stable, and are likely to grab electrons from intact cell membranes. Once they have stolen an electron to balance themselves out, however, the source of that electron is often transformed into a free radical itself. This is how free-radical chain reactions begin, and these kinds of chain reactions would cause significant damage were it not for the existence of antioxidants.

(The body's electron transport chain, which will be described later, also plays a role in controlling oxidative stress, or free-radical damage.)

Antioxidants are nutrients (including vitamins A, C, E, beta-carotene, flavonoids, isoflavones, selenium, and coenzyme Q_{10}) or substances produced in the body (including alpha-lipoic acid and glutathione) that exchange electrons with free radicals. Once it has acquired or released the unpaired electron, the free radical in question is safely neutralized.

Cancer initiation does not mean that a diagnosis of cancer is inevitable. The immune system knows how to recognize and eliminate cancerous cells. Every person's body contains some cells that have undergone cancerous changes. A number of factors influence how quickly these cells multiply. In many cases of prostate cancer, for example, cancer cells multiply so slowly that no treatment is necessary other than "watchful waiting." Different types of cancer multiply at different rates, and a slower-growing tumor may morph into a faster-growing one in response to environmental or internal factors. Multiplying cancer cells invade and obstruct needed space and nutrients. They gum up the works of organ systems and block circulation in the process.

Compared with normal cells, cancer cells use little energy because they are adapted to a less efficient type of metabolism. Two types of metabolism—the process by which sugars, fats, and proteins are "burned" as fuel in the cells' metabolic machinery and turned into energy—exist in the cells of most life forms that require oxygen. There is aerobic (requiring oxygen) metabolism, an intricate biochemical process that leads to the net formation of thirty-eight units of energy and some water. There is also anaerobic metabolism (without oxygen), which nets only two units of energy per unit of fuel. Cancer cells rely on anaerobic metabolism, also known as glycolysis.

TUMOR FORMATION

If the cancer initiation is not stopped, groups of damaged, undifferentiated cells grow together. Once enough cells have been produced from divisions of the initial cancerous cell, a tumor is detectable. Tumors can be benign or malignant. Benign tumors may divide to form enormous masses (for example, uterine fibroids), but they do not invade surrounding normal tissues. They are rarely life threatening. Malignant tumors are made up of individual cells, cords of cells, and nests of cells that invade tissues and spread into organs, blood, and the lymph system. These ever-enlarging groups of cells are no longer under the influence of the normal cell controls. Some cancers take many years to grow large enough to cause physical symptoms; a breast tumor that is detected in a fifty-year-old woman may have begun to form a decade before.

Once a tumor grows large enough to develop its own blood vessels—a process known as angiogenesis—it may sometimes "pinch off" small groups of tumor cells that then float through the lymph system to lodge and grow in other areas of the body. This process is called "metastasis" and is a signpost of a cancer that will ultimately be more difficult to treat.

STANDARD THERAPIES FOR CANCER

Once a cancer is discovered, the usual approach of mainstream oncologists involves one or more of three strategies:

1. Surgically removing the tumor;

2. Giving chemotherapeutic drugs that are designed to target any cancerous cells that remain; and

3. Giving targeted radiation therapy in the area that was affected by cancer in hopes of catching any cancer cells that have escaped the scalpel or the drugs.

Many cancer patients also receive high doses of steroid drugs such as prednisone for the control of edema (fluid buildup) and inflammation. While controlling the inflammatory reaction, this can lead to devastating side effects, as well.

Most of the effort behind the war on cancer has focused on these three treatment modalities—in addition to instruments for early detection, such as mammograms, Pap smears, and prostate-specific antigen (PSA) testing. Cancer therapies have come a very long way since their earliest days. Never before have these cancer treatments been so able to precisely target cancerous growths and spare healthy cells. The efforts of the cancer research community have not been for naught.

Still, chemotherapeutic drugs are highly toxic. They are designed to target rapidly dividing cells, and so often the cells of the body that divide the quickest—including those at the roots of hair and teeth and in the lining of the gastrointestinal tract—may also be attacked. Nausea, vomiting, diarrhea, hair loss, and tooth loss are frequent side effects. In addition to extreme fatigue and anemia resulting from the harsh chemical destruction of the cells, the patient's immunity suffers and the cancer patient can now be vulnerable to life-threatening infections.

Surgeries are often necessary to remove tumors, but cancer cells can be left behind, where they multiply and form a new tumor. Radiation therapy is used to try to "clean up" any remaining cancerous cells following surgery, or may be used when tumors cannot be dealt with surgically. Unfortunately, radiation is a potent carcinogen itself and can cause painful skin burns in cancer patients.

THE DEVELOPMENT OF SAFER CANCER TREATMENTS

Those who research and provide mainstream cancer treatments are trying to work within the U.S. Food and Drug Administration (FDA) guidelines to develop better, safer treatments that attempt to extend life and eliminate cancer from the body. This field has been making improvements in the delivery of targeted chemotherapy and radiation that attempts to limit the destruction of healthy cells while destroying cancer cells. Meanwhile, the field of complementary and alternative cancer medicine continues to expand. Growing numbers of cancer patients are turning to complementary and alternative treatments either to avoid the cut-and-burn approach of mainstream oncology, to ameliorate the negative side effects of chemotherapy and radiation, or to enhance a mainstream approach. Complementary/alternative medicine (CAM) cancer treatments can be seen as clear alternatives to allopathic approaches or they can be viewed as an adjuvant approach to be used along with more mainstream methods.

Alternative cancer medicine seeks less toxic ways to treat cancer. It makes use of a holistic view of this disease, and tries to figure out what tools the body needs to reverse the growth of tumors, while minimizing collateral damage.

Recent groundbreaking research into a specific class of compounds—palladium lipoic compounds—is revealing that they may become the centerpiece of nontoxic cancer therapy. The stories of people who have used these compounds are nothing less than amazing. You'll hear from these people a little later in the book. Now, read on to learn about Poly-MVA and palladium lipoic compounds in general, and about their role in the healing and prevention of cancer.

3. The Story of Poly-MVA

Dr. Merrill Garnett is a research chemist and dentist. He is head of the Garnett McKeen Laboratories in Islip and Bohemia, New York. For the past forty years, Dr. Garnett has researched molecular and cellular biology in order to find effective, nontoxic cancer treatments.

Dr. Garnett began with the research of German scientist Otto Warburg, who was awarded the Nobel Prize for his discovery that cancerous tumors are oxygen deficient and rely upon anaerobic metabolism for energy production. Anaerobic (without oxygen) metabolism produces less energy per unit of fuel, which means decreased energy efficiency in tumor cells. Although these cells are less efficient, this shift is believed to be a form of cellular energy conservation, because less energy is produced.

Dr. Garnett looked at this research and asked: If changes in gene expression alter cellular metabolism in this way, could this be used to somehow target cancerous cells for destruction while leaving healthy cells (those that still utilize primarily aerobic metabolism) alone? Could this decreased energy production be a result of natural selection, where mutant cells that are better able to conserve energy are the ones that survive and multiply? His research focused on ways to identify the enzyme and energy changes that cause the shift from aerobic to anaerobic metabolism, and finding ways to prevent it. Dr. Garnett sought to find a way to utilize the anaerobic energy default mechanism used by cancer cells to bring about their demise.

THE PRODUCT OF DR. GARNETT'S SEARCH

In his book *First Pulse,* Dr. Garnett describes how he searched for "the signaling mechanism by which cells migrate together to form tissues and organs. The cancer cell state is a single cell type of behavior; cancer cells do not form tissues and organs. The organizing communications are missing." In other words, Dr. Garnett sought to discover the signal that tells cells when to form tissues and organs; in so doing, he hoped to discover why cancer cells lack this signal, and how to correct this. By understanding the course of events that triggers the formation and differentiation of normal cells, Dr. Garnett hoped to discover ways to restore these normal events to cancerous cells. "How are these communications interrupted?" Dr. Garnett asked.

In the course of his research, he saw that cancer cells were not malicious entities, but simply immature, or undifferentiated, cells. He sought to discover an enzyme (a substance that catalyzes the activity of biochemical machinery) that would trigger the electron oxygen pathway in order to provide the conditions used by DNA to process developmental changes. He hypothesized that just such an enzyme was missing in cancer cells. By replacing it, he hoped to trigger both the maturation of normal cells and the destruction of these immature, undifferentiated cells.

After more than twenty years of research and laboratory testing with more than 20,000 compounds, Dr. Garnett developed a synthetic enzyme that could facilitate a sort of "selective electrocution" of tumor cells by shuttling electrons into the mitochondria and DNA. This enzyme appeared to be able to target cells that relied upon anaerobic metabolism—cancerous cells— while leaving normal cells intact. Most of the compounds tested were metallo-organic compounds; that is, metals bonded to organic compounds. He sought one that could predictably be toxic to cancerous cells.

Dr. Garnett's rationale for choosing to test specific compounds had to do with complex scientific theories regarding the electrochemical charges he found in DNA and in cells. In fact, his research gave rise to an entirely new field of study called electrogenetics, which studies the energy reactions by which the living state interacts with its hereditary material, DNA. In other words, Dr. Garnett discovered that electrochemical energy is an important "language" used by DNA to communicate with the cell in which it resides, and that this energy is also used for intercellular communication.

Dr. Garnett's electrogenetic theories are backed by highly sensitive electronic studies. Other scientists have studied this electrical genetic pulse, but no other scientist has so deeply delved into its implications, especially for the treatment of cancer. Through the use of sensitive instruments, Dr. Garnett found and was able to measure, beneath the pulse of the heart and all living tissue, a cellular pulse—a vibration that distinguishes the living from the dead, healthy cells from abnormal cells. Dr. Garnett believes that the difference between life and death in the cell and the body is the transfer or movement of electrical energy through the cells and their DNA, which contains all our genes.

Cellular metabolism is, in the end, an electrochemical process. When glucose enters a cell, it is broken down into a substance called acetyl-coA, which is then channeled into a process known as the Krebs cycle, or citric acid cycle. This cycle does not occur in anaerobic metabolism, which is a more primitive form of energy production. The Krebs cycle uses acetyl-coA to produce a high-energy substance known as nicotinamide adenine dinu-cleotide (NADH), which is then oxidized—it donates an electron in a part of the metabolic process called the electron transport chain.

The energy is released along the electron transport chain in the form of voltage jumps. That electrochemical energy is captured in reactions that pre-serve it in the form of adenosine triphosphate (ATP), the energy currency of the body. Any energy needs on the part of the body are filled by the splitting of ATP into adenosine diphosphate (ADP) and a free phosphate molecule.

Dr. Garnett believed that electron transfer somehow held the key to understanding the genetic signaling that would transform cancer cells into healthy ones. He sought to create a sort of "liquid transistor" consisting of a metal and an organic compound (hence, a metallo-organic compound). This liquid transistor would act as an enzyme and affect the electron transfer to DNA. Because of the unique biochemical and electrical properties of metals when bound to organic compounds, he believed that this would be the key. He was right, but it took decades for him to find the right combination. Thousands of biological molecules and several dozen metals fell into the cat-egory of good candidates for such a compound.

Eventually, after over thirty years of research, he struck pay dirt. A spe-cific combination of the metal palladium and the organic molecule alpha-lipoic acid proved to rapidly and efficiently transfer electron charge to DNA. When palladium is sequestered in alpha-lipoic acid, it is benign—useful, in fact—to healthy cells, but for reasons that are not entirely clear, it is toxic to cancer cells. The B vitamin thiamine was also added to create a molecule with a unique structure.

Experiments with cell cultures and mice with cancerous tumors indi-cated that the palladium–alpha-lipoic acid–thiamine compound was toxic to cancer cells but had no adverse effects on healthy cells. One day, in the early 1990s, the laboratory mice treated with this compound stopped dying from their once-fatal form of cancer, and analysis showed that the compound was selectively eliminating cancerous cells.

This is how palladium lipoic complexes (LAPd) were created. Dr. Garnett took out several patents on this class of compounds. One form is currently in the preclinical preparation for the pharmaceutical-approval process. Another form, Poly-MVA, is available as a nutritional supplement.

THANKS TO DR. AL SANCHEZ . . .

The story of Poly-MVA would not be complete without mention of the tireless commitment of Al Sanchez Sr., Ed.S., Ph.D. Dr. Sanchez lost his wife to colon cancer in 1972, when she was only thirty-four years old. At the time, he was working as a school principal, but the course of his life shifted dramatically after his wife's death. He vowed to spend the rest of his life searching for effective nontoxic treatments for cancer. He sought out substances that had some scientific support as cancer fighters, using his considerable "people skills" to network with those who research and create natural cancer remedies. As long as the evidence showed that they would not cause harm, he gave them to advanced-cancer patients to try.

His diligent searching paid off when he came across Dr. Garnett and Poly-MVA. After reviewing the research and earlier success of the product, Dr. Sanchez purchased Poly-MVA for distribution to cancer patients. To his delight and astonishment, success stories began flooding in, some of which are included in Chapter 7.

Dr. Sanchez's approach is diametrically opposed to that of mainstream medical science. Most conventional physicians are unlikely to recommend a compound to their patients if it has not undergone rigorous, extensive clinical testing that proves its safety and efficacy and brings it FDA approval. On the other hand, if one can prove that something is safe and completely nontoxic, and there is convincing evidence in its favor along with a solid scientific basis, it's worth trying, especially for people who are dying of cancer. Poly-MVA and other palladium lipoic complexes fall into this category of alternative cancer therapies.

It's true that clinical studies—the kind needed for FDA approval of a drug—are required. Many are underway. Some would argue that we must not recommend any substance that hasn't undergone this stringent and enormously costly process, especially if we don't exactly understand how that substance does what it is purported to do. The truth is, however, that aspirin was used for many years before anyone knew how it worked. Throughout history, herbal and natural medicines have been used successfully without any scientific analysis of their direct effects on human physiology.

Most clinical testing attempts to isolate the effects of a single substance on disease. One common criticism of alternative cancer remedies is that they haven't been tested alone—that is, without dietary changes or the addition of other supplements and/or drugs. However, it is hardly fair to expect people who are dying from cancer to try only one intervention at a time. Disease is a multifactorial process, and so must be the treatment of disease—especially a disease as complex and dangerous as cancer. Eventually Poly-MVA will probably be studied as a sole remedy for cancer, but for now, it makes sense for cancer patients to use any and all dietary changes, nutritional supplements, and medical methods at their disposal to improve their chances of a cure.

Dr. Sanchez established the nonprofit company the Foundation for Advancement in Cancer Research, with the intention of getting the word out about alternative cancer therapies, including Poly-MVA. Slowly, the word is spreading. If you were to do an Internet search for Poly-MVA, you would find dozens of articles, scientific information, more inspiring stories of cancer survival, and further information about Dr. Merrill Garnett's research and discovery.

4. Understanding Poly-MVA

A biochemist working in the Biochemistry and Cell Biology lab at a leading northeastern university appreciated the brilliance of Dr. Garnett's electrogenetic theories about palladium lipoic complexes, but saw the need for an explanation of its actions from the perspective of cellular and molecular biology. This kind of explanation would give the research community and physicians a more concrete understanding of how these compounds could be used to heal cancer.

A report by this biochemist provided strong support for the anti-carcinogenic action of palladium lipoic complexes (LAPds) through a mechanism that no other scientist had yet elucidated. He found that LAPds can selectively target and kill tumor cells through changes in the action of an enzyme called pyruvate dehydrogenase (PDH).

Highly developed complex organisms use oxygen (aerobic metabolism) to provide extra energy for complex processes and movement. Anaerobic metabolism, which takes place without oxygen, is used by the ancient forms of life like bacteria living in areas devoid of oxygen. PDH is the bridge between anaerobic and aerobic metabolism. In healthy, unstressed cells, anaerobic and aerobic metabolism occur in sequence. As shown in Figure 1 on page 16, during anaerobic metabolism, glucose is broken down into pyruvate, a 3-carbon substance, without the use of oxygen. The breaking of the bonds of glucose to create pyruvate yields two units of adenosine triphosphate (ATP)—the body's energy currency. The enzyme PDH creates a bridge between anaerobic metabolism (glycolysis) and the Krebs cycle (aerobic metabolism). The pyruvate molecules are channeled into aerobic metabolism. The electron transport chain is part of the Krebs cycle, and combined, these two processes yield thirty-eight units of ATP. Without PDH, the final step of glycolytic energy production cannot take place, and the cell shifts to primarily anaerobic metabolism.

PDH activity is altered in cancerous cells, and it is believed by some that

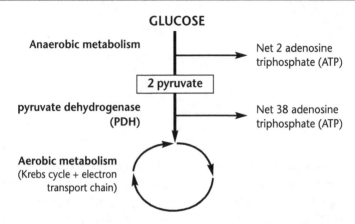

FIGURE 1. A simplified view of the breakdown of glucose (carbohydrate) into energy during cellular metabolism.

LAPds work by affecting PDH. This is believed to eliminate the primary means of ATP production (anaerobic metabolism) within tumor cells, and, in so doing, cellular process crucial to the growth and long-term survival of the cell is inhibited.

WHAT IS POLY-MVA?

Poly-MVA is a patented palladium lipoic compound, one of several palladium lipoic complexes (LAPds). The initials "MVA" stand for "minerals, vitamins, and amino acids." Promising evidence indicates that its ingredients can target and eliminate cancerous cells without harming healthy ones by affecting PDH and/or altering DNA energy transfer patterns that appear to be associated with malignant transformation.

It's easy to see that while Poly-MVA's most important use is in the battle against cancer, its total lack of toxicity and its many rejuvenating and healing effects on cell function make it an ideal cellular nutrient for prevention of other diseases and support of optimal health and quality of life. See Chapter 8 for more on the use of Poly-MVA for support of optimal health.

Poly-MVA is a proprietary formulation that contains palladium, alpha-lipoic acid, vitamins B_1, B_2, and B_{12}, the amino acids formyl-methionine and acetylcysteine, and trace amounts of the metals molybdenum, rhodium, and ruthenium. Each ingredient has its own unique characteristics and healing properties, as follows.

Palladium

Palladium is a unique and rare metal that has special properties. In Poly-MVA, it is sequestered in an organic molecule called alpha-lipoic acid and provides the unique electrochemical, electron-transferring aspect that makes the compound so revolutionary.

Alpha-Lipoic Acid (ALA)

Alpha-lipoic acid (ALA) is one of the most powerful antioxidants and detoxifiers known to humanity. It is soluble in both fat and water, and readily crosses membranes throughout the body, particularly when bound to palladium. It can pass through the virtually impenetrable blood-brain barrier—a characteristic that makes this nutrient ideal for moving the other components of Poly-MVA into brain cells to help heal brain cancer.

The importance of ALA in biological systems has been known since the 1950s. It is made within the body, and is a necessary part of cellular metabolism. It has powerful antioxidant capacity, but only acts as an antioxidant when supplemental amounts are available to the cells. In other words, ALA made by the body has important work to do in the energy factories of the cells, and none of it can be spared for antioxidant work unless ALA is brought in from outside the body. However, only tiny amount of ALA can be found in most foods.

When enough ALA is available, it helps to directly deactivate free radicals. It also donates electrons to other antioxidants that have "spent" themselves doing the same kind of work. Alpha-lipoic acid also regenerates vitamin E, vitamin C, and glutathione. Glutathione is an antioxidant that is made in the body. It is a powerful cellular detoxifier, especially in the liver. People with cancer, autoimmune disease, AIDS, and other diseases have been found to have low levels of glutathione. ALA is the only antioxidant that's been proven to raise glutathione levels within the cells.

ALA also inhibits glycation, the process by which sugars bind to proteins within cells. When you watch a chicken browning in the oven, you're observing glycation in action. Age spots on the skin are another visible manifestation of glycation. This process is believed to be an important cause of premature aging and age-related disease. Glycated proteins produce free radicals at a rate fifty times that of non-glycated proteins.

ALA is also an effective chelator of heavy metals. It helps to move excessive amounts of metals such as mercury, iron, and copper safely out of the body. These are metals that catalyze (enhance) the production of free radicals when allowed to accumulate in excess.

Several recent studies indicate that ALA is extremely helpful for the treatment of diabetic complications (such as nerve damage in the extremities and the eyes) and may aid in the prevention of Parkinson's disease and Alzheimer's disease. ALA may even be involved in nerve regeneration.

B Vitamins

The B vitamins act as coenzymes in the process of cellular respiration. Vitamin B_1 (thiamine) is involved in the decarboxylation (the removal of a carboxyl group—a carbon, two oxygen, and a hydrogen) of pyruvate and the oxidation of alpha keto-glutamic acid, two of the reactions of the Krebs cycle. These functions are essential for energy production, carbohydrate metabolism, and neurotransmitter function. Extreme deficiency of vitamin B_1 is rare in most developed countries, but mild deficiency can cause fatigue, depression, tingling or numbness in the extremities, and constipation.

Vitamin B_2 (riboflavin) is also a coenzyme. It is required for cellular metabolism, as part of the flavin adenine dinucleotide (FAD) and flavin mononucleotide (FMN) Krebs cycle systems. FAD and FMN are involved in the production of two crucial antioxidants, glutathione peroxidase and xanthine oxidase, and are important parts of the cytochrome 450 detoxification system, the liver's primary route for detoxifying potentially harmful substances.

Along with folic acid, vitamin B_{12} (cobalamin) is involved in DNA synthesis, in the production of the myelin sheaths that protect nerves and improve their conductivity, and in the production of red blood cells. Vitamin B_{12} is one of the vitamins needed to lower levels of the amino acid homocysteine, which in excess is toxic to blood vessel walls and is now known to be a major cause of deadly cardiovascular disease. The digestive factors in the stomach needed to absorb vitamin B_{12} decrease with age, and this is why B_{12} deficiency is quite common in people over age sixty-five. In fact, a deficiency in vitamin B_{12} is often an underlying cause of short-term memory loss that is mistaken for the early signs of dementia. One study found that 61 percent of patients with vitamin B_{12} deficiency showed marked improvements in mental capacity with the use of B_{12} supplements.

Formyl-methionine

Formyl-methionine is a form of the sulfur-containing amino acid methionine. It is used as the first amino acid to build a protein. As precursor to cysteine (discussed below), it is needed to make the antioxidant glutathione. Most important, methionine participates in a process known as methylation, in which methyl groups are added to compounds. This action of methionine aids liver detoxification and is believed to help prevent DNA changes that can lead to cancer initiation.

N-acetylcysteine (NAC)

N-acetylcysteine (NAC) is a naturally occurring antioxidant amino acid, a form of cysteine. Its antioxidant potency is well established in scientific literature, and like ALA, it helps to boost the action of other antioxidants, including vitamins C and E. Studies show that supplemental NAC enhances immunity, improves lung function, helps in the transport of certain hormones, and helps prevent insulin resistance.

Molybdenum

Molybdenum is an essential trace mineral that is crucial for the regulation of pH (a measure of acidity or alkalinity) in the body. Cancerous cells are depleted of oxygen, and they also tend to be excessively acidic. Anaerobic metabolism produces acid. If you're a workout buff, you may know that when you "go for the burn" with high-intensity exercise, you're producing a lot of lactic acid that builds up in your muscles—and cells that are overly acidic are cells that are stressed out.

Rhodium and Ruthenium

Rhodium is a rare earth metal that is noted for its low electrical resistance and high corrosion resistance, and is used as a catalyst for many chemical processes. Ruthenium is another transition metal of the platinum group that is used to harden and increase the corrosion resistance of titanium. It is also a versatile catalyst. It is interesting to note that ruthenium/molybdenum alloys have been found to be superconductive.

HOW POLY-MVA WORKS

Two mechanisms for the anticancer effects of Poly-MVA have been proposed: Merrill Garnett's electrogenetic theory and the pyruvate dehydrogenase theory mentioned at the start of this chapter.

Dr. Garnett's electrogenetic theories are described in Chapter 3. These theories have been peer-reviewed and published, but a thorough understanding of electrogenetic theory requires multidisciplinary training in chemistry, biology, and physics. Dr. Garnett's findings are difficult to disseminate to laypersons in a form that is both understandable and scientifically accurate. They are, however, indispensable for a comprehensive picture of how Poly-MVA functions.

The PDH theory of how Poly-MVA works is based in molecular biology, but the electrochemical charges described by Dr. Garnett play an important role in this explanation. Both electrogenetics and molecular biology are necessary to explain the effects of this compound on cancer cells.

In laboratory studies designed to test the PDH theory, the predictable death of cancer cells within twenty-four hours following their exposure to LAPd turned out to hinge upon the lab's decision to purchase inexpensive glass slides that are made with silicates:

When added to a cancer cell culture, LAPd causes cancer cells to stop growing within eighteen hours—but only if the slide used to make the culture is made of glass. This is because the inexpensive glass used to make slides contains silicates, which lend the glass an electrical charge; this charge activates the LAPd's effects on the cancer cells' DNA. Then, the cells become slightly rounded, remain alive for about twenty-four hours, and then become almost spherical. They detach from their source of nourishment (a substrate added to the cell culture to keep the cancer cells alive while they are being studied) and gradually die.

The finding that the charge of the slide plays such an important role in the ability of LAPd to kill cancer cells seems, at first glance, to be a problem—until it is recognized that tumor cells have a deficit in electrical charge flow when compared with normal cells! This partly explains how the LAPd compound targets and electrocutes cancer cells. (F. J. Antonawich, S. M. Fiore, J. N. David, 1998.)

Poly-MVA is a very promising alternative therapy for cancer. It is presently being used as an adjunct treatment for cancer by numerous physicians and other healthcare practitioners around the world. Its use is becoming increasingly widespread as doctors and patients see firsthand how the product of Dr. Garnett's decades of work can save lives and positively affect people's health when used as part of a comprehensive nutritional program for cancer therapy.

5. Energy Medicine: Bridging East and West

While great strides have been made in Western medicine for treating certain types of illnesses such as infectious diseases and surgical disorders, the prevention and treatment of chronic disorders with Western medicines remains poor. The biochemical model is very limited when trying to treat disease syndromes and chronic disease and focuses on the pathologic degeneration of a condition—ignoring the mind-body connection and the existence of energy fields. It is in these energetic fields where disturbances are first manifested. Because of this disparity between what is perceived and the reality of medical care satisfaction, doctors and patients alike argue over the possible solutions for their medical problems. Just as in the ancient times where there was a strong dialogue between Asclepios, god of medicine, and Hygeia, goddess of health, today a new dialogue, a new language is being developed to begin to understand the concept of bioenergy as part of the holistic concept of the treating the whole body, mind, and spirit.

Manning and Vanrenen noted in their book *Bioenergetic Medicine East and West,*

> "On the surface the mechanical, biochemical model of Western medicine is mathematical, neat and tidy, but the dynamic, chaotic nature of life and of man tends to undermine this semblance of order. Modern science has striven to make medicine into a hard science like chemistry and to avoid the unquantifiable the: emotions, spirit and subjective sensations. The monumental effort drive to make medicine into a consistent, hard science solely based on biochemical data, tends to disregard the traditional art of healing based on homeostasis and bioenergy" (C. Manning, L. Vanrenen, 1988, p. 24).

The essential distinction between the biochemical model of Western medicine and Eastern medicine is the concept of energy and energy flow—the recognition of the unseen, subatomic world in dynamic action. As Dr.

Larry Dossey explained in *Space, Time, and Medicine*, "In the first place, as the physicist Wheeler has observed, 'the world is at the bottom a quantum world and quantum system' " (L. Dossey, p. 146). This means that we will ultimately give due regard to the subatomic world. In an article in *Foundation of Physics*, physicist David Bohm noted, "we see the universe that the insepa-rable quantum interconnectedness of the whole universe is the fundamental reality, and that the relatively behaving parts are merely particular and con-tingent within the whole" (D. Bohm, 1975).

The holistic perspective involves the understanding of bioenergy, home-ostasis, and the integrity of the whole. Each individual person is considered a unique ecological system vitalized and regulated by bioenergy. Over the past twenty-five years, there has been increasing Western interest in the holistic studies and Eastern medical approaches such as acupuncture, Chinese medi-cine, Ayurvedic medicine, and homeopathy. These "old" medical systems are each based on the bioenergetic nature of diagnosis and treatment. In health, the bioenergy of the patient is balanced and strong. In dis-ease, an interfer-ence or weakness overcomes the normal vibration rate of the bioenergy, caus-ing distortions in the energy field. These are called patterns of disharmony and are unique characteristics of bioenergetic medicine.

The science of the future will include the vigorous methodology of sci-ence as well as an integrated understanding of the whole.

When Dr. Garnett describes the electrical charge characteristics of DNA, he uses an elegant combination of the languages of physics, chemistry, and Eastern medicine. Although it may seem overwhelmingly complex, DNA car-ries an electrical (thus bioenergetic) charge.

"When two polymers are associated with hyaluronic acid, they each form cables microscopically resembling the parallel twin wire trans-mission cables used in electronics. Such transmission cables are effi-cient for signal transfer at defined electronic impedance, voltage, and frequency. I have reported that these paired polymers produce an inductance field when they are exposed to a pulsed cation current. This is in keeping with the Faraday Maxwell Law of Induction as in wires, coils, and transformers. A model for cell DNA-to-cell DNA inductive signaling is suggested by the intermediate role of pro-thrombin-hyaluronic acid acting with the coil-to-coil field geometry of an electric transformer. The vascular flow of prothrombin then forms a kind of common biological Internet for cells to log on to. Hence, tissue synchronization" (Garnett, www.electrogenetics.com).

We can quickly see that there is a new language being developed in the sciences to understand what has heretofore been unthinkable: Energy production. Energy transfer. Energy blockage. Energy dissipation—in the human body!

Thanks to Dr. Garnett and his colleagues, there will soon be a scientific understanding of "energy," and the lines of demarcation between East and West medicine will begin to disappear.

For now, suffice to say that there are doctors and acupuncturists who are using Poly-MVA to enhance the flow of energy or "Chi." Once they understood that Poly-MVA is a bioenergetic catalyst for the transfer of energy, these innovative practitioners have found that acupuncture energy transfer is enhanced when they use acupuncture needles dipped in Poly-MVA or diluted Poly-MVA injected into acupuncture points. Energy transfer is sustained for a significantly longer time than insertion of needles alone. The author (Robert D. Milne, M.D.) feels that further research will document the salutary effects of this special use for Poly-MVA.

6. Poly-MVA: Research Evidence

This chapter includes a summary of the laboratory research that has been done to explain Poly-MVA's apparent effectiveness in supporting health and healing cancer. Oncological surgeon Rudolf E. Falk presented the first report of clinical studies of Poly-MVA at the Adjuvant Nutrition in Cancer Treatment Symposium in March 1994. In his work at the University of Toronto, Dr. Falk administered Poly-MVA intravenously to ninety-five patients. The cancers from which these patients suffered included cancers of the breast, lung, colon, rectum, prostate, pancreas, ovary, skin (malignant melanoma), and brain. Ninety percent of these patients had failed to improve after undergoing virtually all available therapy.

During their experimental treatment with Poly-MVA, they received moderate doses of chemotherapy. Under normal circumstances, 20 to 60 percent of such patients would only survive an average of another six months. However, nine months after initiation of intravenous Poly-MVA, 90 percent of them were still alive.

ROUTE OF ADMINISTRATION

Poly-MVA is most often taken orally, as it was designed to be used. Does Poly-MVA have to be given intravenously to have the effect described in Dr. Falk's report? Although the research has yet to answer this question, we have no reason to believe that the usual way of taking this supplement (as a liquid mixed with water or juice) would not be as effective. Some physicians who offer Poly-MVA therapy to their patients choose to give it intravenously, specifically when they are treating end-stage cancer patients. Many are also combining intravenous Poly-MVA with oxidative therapies such as ozone therapy and hydrogen peroxide therapy.

All of the components of Poly-MVA are absorbed through the walls of the gastrointestinal tract. Patients who take it orally—and this includes most of the patients who have tried it—report good results. Intravenous use moves the nutrients to the cells more quickly, but the research is not there yet to support widespread intravenous use of Poly-MVA. The lipoic acid complexes were designed by Dr. Garnett for oral use, and for now—until more research evidence has come back from labs and physicians who are using it in IV form—it's best to stick with the oral-dosing regimen, which has been in use since 1995.

POLY-MVA AND GLIOBLASTOMA

Pharmakon Laboratories performed animal studies to determine the safety and effectiveness of palladium lipoic complexes (LAPds) in the treatment of glioblastoma, a fast-growing and highly dangerous brain cancer. At the beginning of the study, glioblastoma tumor cells were injected into the scruff of the neck of Swiss nude mice. When tumors had grown to 200–400 millimeters in volume, the mice were divided into eight groups of ten. Four groups were given daily intravenous doses of either LAPd or placebo; four groups were given intraperitoneal doses (tube feeding) of either LAPd or placebo. Those who were given LAPd received doses of 1.5, 1, or 2 milligrams per mouse for a total of four weeks, and tumor volume was monitored throughout. Mice that died were dissected and tumor volume was compared between groups. Not surprisingly, the mice that received the LAPd had significantly reduced growth of the glioblastoma tumor cell line. All of the intravenously treated mice showed significant reduction in tumor size compared with placebo. Of the mice given LAPd through tube feeding, dosages of 1 to 2 milligrams per mouse—a dose comparable to that used in humans with cancer—had significant effects, shrinking tumor size.

Frank Antonawich, Ph.D., is a neurobiology professor at the State University of New York at Stony Brook. His study (coauthored by S. M. Fiore and J. N. Davis), "The Effects of a Lipoic Acid/Palladium Complex on Hippocampal Progenitor Cells," was published in abstract form by the Society for Neuroscience in 1998. His work is based on preliminary research and anecdotal reports showing that LAPd may be an effective anti-glioblastoma agent. Immortalized hippocampal cells—cells that multiply out of control much like cancerous cells do—were cultured on specially coated (electrically charged) plates and plastic plates. Cells cultured on plastic, which holds no charge, were completely unaffected by the LAPd, but those on the specially coated plates were killed by the compound. Professor Antonawich has continued his research and at the time of this writing has submitted further papers on the benefits and uses of Poly-MVA and palladium lipoic complexes.

Despite the minimal amount of peer-reviewed evidence on the clinical efficacy of LAPd in the treatment of any condition, there is a reasonable amount of safety data, clinical application, and solid scientific information, which is available for independent research, to justify its use as an adjunct cancer treatment. The extent of LAPd's effectiveness or what agents may be used in conjunction with it to have an optimum effect are unknown at this time because of the multiple variables associated with this disease and the need for further research that is currently underway.

HOW SAFE ARE POLY-MVA AND OTHER PALLADIUM LIPOIC COMPLEXES?

The results of toxicology studies in animals show that LAPd and Poly-MVA are very safe and nontoxic. No deaths or signs of organ damage occurred in test animals that were given extremely high doses. It was concluded that the LD50 (the dose lethal to 50 percent of test animals) of LAPd exceeds 5,000 milligrams per kilogram of body weight. The average human dose is 6 milligrams per kilogram of body weight per day.

The only risk factor that has been observed with LAPd in high doses is in patients with significant cancerous lesions in the lungs who are at risk of pleural effusion (collection of fluid in the lungs). Several cases have been reported in which LAPd was administered to such patients, and the fluid in their lungs increased. The available information on LAPd's action indicates that this may be the result of a "die-off" of malignant cells, which can cause a variety of unpleasant symptoms as the body works to eliminate them through the detoxification pathways. Patients who fit this description should be observed while using Poly-MVA.

7. True Stories of Cancer Survival with Poly-MVA

This chapter contains true stories from real cancer patients who have used palladium lipoic complexes. These stories have been collected from the Poly-MVA Survivors' website, from the *Townsend Letter for Doctors & Patients* magazine, and from the files of the Association for Wholintegral Medicine, Inc.

Almost every person whose story you will read here made drastic changes in his or her diet and lifestyle, and many used various other nutritional supplements, in an effort to heal themselves of cancer. The common denominator in their stories of renewed health, however, is the use of Poly-MVA. Some had been using other natural methods to try to heal their cancers, but didn't experience significant pain relief or disease regression until they added Poly-MVA to their regimens.

In several cases, the patient's success with Poly-MVA and other holistic therapies has been considerable enough to convince even skeptical mainstream medical practitioners to look into this nontoxic method for healing cancer.

HARRY QUICK, D.V.M.

After being diagnosed with adenocarcinoma in 2002, Harry Quick, D.V.M., had a cancerous lesion removed from beneath his left armpit. Doctors recommended radiation treatment, but Dr. Quick refused and sought out "an alternative, less destructive protocol." He used a Japanese product called MGN-3 to enhance the activity of the immune cells responsible for singling out and destroying cancerous cells. Unfortunately, within two weeks after his surgery, his tumor returned, and a month later, it was the size of a golf ball. He knew he needed to do something, and fast.

After some thorough research, Dr. Quick determined that he needed to make a lot of lifestyle changes, including modifying his eating habits and avoiding toxins. He controlled his stress level and began to exercise regularly, and made a greater effort to participate in his community. He also took massive doses of intravenous vitamin C. For three hours a day, he sat with an IV line in his arm, dripping 75,000 grams of vitamin C into his bloodstream. By June's end, his tumor was the size of a pea, but he suspected that the vitamin C treatments were dehydrating his body, and he wanted to seek out something else. He then began to use Poly-MVA.

After two weeks of taking 12 teaspoons of Poly-MVA a day, Dr. Quick sent his blood plasma to a lab for an AMAS test, which is used to measure anti-malignan antibodies, a marker of whether the immune system is actively destroying cancer cells. For the following thirty days, he took 6 teaspoons of Poly-MVA a day along with coenzyme Q_{10}, MGN-3, a probiotic supplement, multiple vitamins and minerals, and a diet of organic vegetables with some chicken and fish, after which further tests showed him to be in remission, and he was feeling much improved. After a final surge in a subsequent AMAS test (a common result of cancer cell "die-off"), a PET scan and a final AMAS test in November showed that his body was free of cancer.

MARILYN ULREY

This fifty-eight-year-old nurse was given two weeks to live in the summer of 2002. She was under hospice care at that time. About two years earlier, Ms. Ulrey had a double mastectomy, and was advised to have both radiation and chemotherapy. She refused both. Her cancer spread with a vengeance, metastasizing to her brain, skull, legs, and face. Both of her femurs (long bones in the legs) broke because of bone metastases. She was told that she had three different types of cancer, all aggressive. Ms. Ulrey's tumors grew so large that they disfigured her face.

Ms. Ulrey started Poly-MVA on August 26, 2002. She continued to use MGN-3, coral calcium, and coenzyme Q_{10}, as well as the drug clodronate (used to prevent bone metastases) and a liver detoxification program, all of which she had been using throughout the course of her disease. After ninety-six days on 8 teaspoons of Poly-MVA a day, her husband noticed a very strong body odor and rashes on the tumors on her head and face. Eventually, Ms. Ulrey regained her ability to walk (with a walker) and to do daily activities, and she had begun to work out for two hours each day to strengthen her legs. She also regained her ability to think, write, cook, and speak as her tumors shrank. Her appetite dramatically improved.

On April 15, 2003, Marilyn Ulrey left the hospice program. No other patient had ever gotten well enough to leave the program.

GRACIE TODORCZUK

This forty-two-year-old breast cancer survivor discovered Poly-MVA very shortly after her breast cancer diagnosis on January 24, 2001. Her 2.3-centimeter invasive infiltrating ductal carcinoma was removed with a lumpectomy on February 20. She was told that there had been a small area of lymph node invasion. At the time of her surgery, she had been taking Poly-MVA for fifteen days, and a preoperative ultrasound showed that her tumor had shrunk.

Ms. Todorczuk also followed a strict holistic program, starting with her diagnosis. Since her lumpectomy, all follow-up exams have shown her to be cancer-free, without subjecting herself to chemotherapy or radiation. After getting yet another clean bill of health at a follow-up with her surgeon, the surgeon decided to take a careful look at the program that had enabled his patient to go from stage III cancer to cancer-free without toxic therapies.

JOHN MERRITT

This sixty-year-old stockbroker was diagnosed with stage IV glioblastoma multiform in March 2000. This fast-growing brain cancer is notoriously difficult to treat. At Cedars-Sinai Hospital in Los Angeles, Mr. Merritt underwent surgery in April 2000, followed by thirty-three rounds of radiation. His tumor returned, and he had a second surgery in which Gliadel wafers (small plastic discs that contain cancer-killing drugs) were inserted into the cancerous tissue.

An MRI at the end of October showed regrowth. Oncologists recommended the chemotherapy drug vincristine, but Mr. Merritt and his wife had found messages about Poly-MVA at a brain tumor support group website and decided to try it first. He began to take Poly-MVA in November 2000. Since that time, he has continued to work, play golf, and travel. Mrs. Merritt reports that her husband has suffered no memory deficits—she even feels his memory has improved somewhat! An MRI from February 2001 showed that his tumor had decreased in mass. Six months later, Mr. Merritt was continuing to live a full, active life. John had been doing wonderfully, living a full life with no restrictions. In July of 2002 he had another MRI that showed a mass but it was stable. The doctor convinced John to try another chemotherapy and from that time his health diminished until his death in February 2004.

MAUREEN ARNETT

Despite the fact that she has always been health conscious and cancer didn't run in her family, Ms. Arnett had to have her cancerous ascending colon and several lymph nodes removed in May 2002. She recovered quickly from the surgery and was advised to undergo chemotherapy, which she refused. Instead, she began taking Poly-MVA immediately after her surgery, starting with 8 teaspoons a day and dropping down to 4 teaspoons a day after two months. She also took several other supplements for liver detoxification, including freshly pressed wheatgrass juice, a liver-support supplement containing milk thistle, artichoke leaf, dandelion root, turmeric, amino acids, MGN-3, and coenzyme Q_{10}. She also followed a diet tailored to her blood type. Her follow-ups have revealed no cancer anywhere in her body, and she reports feeling great and being active every day.

JOSEPH WHITE

Joseph White had a stroke that caused partial right-side paralysis in 1998. Later, he developed back pain so severe that he could not sleep, and in September 2001 he was diagnosed with prostate cancer that had metastasized to his hip bones. Radiation, surgery to remove the prostate, and chemotherapy were all recommended, but Mr. White decided against all of them. He treated his pain with painkilling medication.

In November of that year, he received some literature on Poly-MVA. His PSA was 225 by then—a score indicative of advanced cancer. He took Poly-MVA for two months, and by January 15, 2002, his PSA had dropped to 5 and his pain had gone away completely. When his doctor saw these results, he was—in the patient's words—"utterly amazed and became a believer himself."

KENNETH WALKER

This sixty-seven-year-old clergyman's story appeared in an article by Morton Walker, D.P.M., printed in the February/March 2003 issue of *Townsend Letter for Doctors & Patients*. Reverend Walker was diagnosed with multiple myeloma—a diffuse cancer that affects bones throughout the body—in March 2001. He had terrible bone pain in his head, ribs, spine, and elsewhere, and when he was diagnosed, physicians found holes in his skull the size of small coins. His oncology team informed him that without chemotherapy, he would have less than three months to live. Multiple myeloma, reports Dr.

Walker (no relation to Reverend Walker) in his article, kills 52 percent of patients within three months of diagnosis, and 90 percent die within three years.

Reverend Walker turned to Poly-MVA for support, and was well enough to spend the late summer of 2001 sailing around Vancouver Island with his wife in their sailboat. More than a year later, he could be found scuba diving in Aruba. He credits much of his recovery to the use of Poly-MVA.

ADDITIONAL CASE STUDIES

Chip White, a researcher with the Association for Wholintegral Medicine (AWM), has more than ten years of experience working with alternative approaches to cancer therapy. Mr. White has been engaged in an extensive analysis of patients who have used Poly-MVA. These case studies provide further insight into the breakthrough results that Poly-MVA, along with other lifestyle changes, has had on the lives of cancer patients.

Case Study 1

A male glioblastoma patient, sixty-six years of age, had convulsions and paralysis of his right leg and foot. Four days after starting Poly-MVA, he reported that his paralysis was gone and he could walk outside, water his lawn, and ride his stationary bicycle. Eight days after starting Poly-MVA, he called to report that his convulsions were occurring less frequently.

Case Study 2

A fifty-six-year-old breast cancer survivor had metastases to her spine and right hip. She received a right hip replacement to gain relief from the pain her cancer had been causing, but still had severe back pain. Within two weeks of starting Poly-MVA, she reported that her back pain had stopped and she was able to return to her job.

Case Study 3

Two patients with cancer of the esophagus required strong pain-relief medication. Both were terminal and had lost an extreme amount of fat and muscle. Patient A, aged sixty-two, was in a hospital in Mexico, and although scheduled to start Poly-MVA, this patient only received laetrile (another alternative cancer therapy), and died shortly after. Patient B, aged forty-five, received the Poly-MVA and soon reported increased strength and weight gain. This patient was still alive two years later.

CASE STUDY 4

An Alaskan woman diagnosed with multiple myeloma sent a letter to the makers of Poly-MVA. She had received her diagnosis in April 1995, and after taking Poly-MVA for a little over two years, she was told that her blood tests and exams showed "no measurable signs of multiple myeloma carcinoma" and that she was "in total remission."

The doses used in the above five cases studies may have been lower than optimal; current research is being conducted with higher dosages. Chip White also reports that colon cancer patients with obstruction report improvements after using Poly-MVA. Poly-MVA's solubility in both fat and water allow it to pass easily through membranes such as the one that lines the large intestine.

MANY MORE SUCCESS STORIES

The happy endings don't end here. There are many other stories of people who have used natural healing modalities along with palladium lipoic complexes to halt or reverse the spread of advanced cancers. Most of these people were told that they were giving themselves a certain death sentence by refusing chemotherapy and radiation.

8. Using Poly-MVA for Nutritional Support and Cancer Therapy

Poly-MVA is a promising alternative therapy for cancer, but it can be used to great advantage in people without cancer. Research by Garnett McKeen Laboratories and others show that Poly-MVA can do the following:

- Aid in cellular energy production.

- Support the liver in the removal of harmful substances from the body.

- Assist in the prevention of cell damage.

- Assist the body in removing heavy metals from the bloodstream.

- Act as a powerful antioxidant, neutralizing free radicals within the cells and utilizing them to make energy.

- Support nerve and neurotransmitter function.

- Enhance white blood cell function.

- Assist in unblocking energy flow in acupuncture meridians.

If you've read this far, you might think that you have to have cancer in order to benefit from Poly-MVA. This is not the case. Although research is not conclusive on this front, what is known so far points to Poly-MVA's having a cancer-preventative effect. If you use a maintenance dose, you would likely be protecting yourself against the growth and spread of cancerous cells before any tumors are detectable. In a time when one out of three people can expect to have cancer at some point, it makes sense to improve your odds every way you can.

The research of Frank Antonawich, Ph.D., has demonstrated that Poly-MVA and other palladium lipoic complexes are useful for the prevention of brain damage following stroke, for the prevention of heart damage following heart attack, and for the treatment of damage related to hypertension. In a talk given on March 29, 2003, Dr. Antonawich spoke about the effects of Poly-MVA on animals subjected to TIA (transient ischemic attack). Normally, the type of TIA used in experimental animals damages the part of the brain that directs the animals' nest-building ability. Some gerbils underwent surgery in which TIA was induced; the control group underwent a benign procedure. Dr. Antonawich reported: "Within 24 hours, behavioral protection was evident. I immediately knew which animals got the drug [Poly-MVA]. My technician was shocked; when I came back in from giving a lecture, I just walked in and said, 'You gave it to numbers 3, 7, 9, and 12.' She said, 'Yeah!' All of them had beautiful nests built."

The animals that had been given the TIA without the Poly-MVA had not been able to build nests. The Poly-MVA had offered 60 to 70 percent protection against TIA-inflicted brain damage; other drugs have been able to achieve only 30 to 40 percent protection.

Dr. Merrill Garnett has also been studying the protective effects of palladium lipoic complexes, looking at their benefits against radiation sickness. (See Garnett and Remo, "DNA Reductase: A Synthetic Enzyme with Opportunist Clinical Activity Against Radiation Sickness," International Symposium on Applications of Enzymes in Chemistry, 2001.)

A novel use of Poly-MVA is the injection of diluted Poly-MVA into acupuncture points. It should be noted that many patients with chronic fatigue and fibromyalgia respond more favorably to acupuncture treatment with Poly-MVA than with acupuncture treatment alone.

POLY-MVA AND AUTOIMMUNE DISEASES

The usual medical treatments for autoimmune diseases, in which the immune system overreacts and creates inflammation somewhere in the body, include chemotherapy drugs and high doses of steroids. These therapies can be more devastating than the disease itself. It appears that Poly-MVA may offer a nontoxic alternative to those who suffer from autoimmune conditions.

Psoriasis is a skin condition that affects more than 7 million Americans. It is believed that it may be caused by autoimmune process. Psoriasis creates itchy, flaky, reddened patches of skin that can be isolated to small areas or can affect almost the entire body. Practitioners who use Poly-MVA have found that given orally and topically it is effective for the treatment of psoriasis—even in the most severe cases. Other autoimmune diseases, including multiple sclerosis and lupus, have also been successfully treated with Poly-MVA. Research is underway for the use of palladium lipoic complexes for auto-immune diseases.

POLY-MVA AND ENDOMETRIOSIS

Endometriosis is a condition that afflicts 10 to 20 percent of all women in the United States. Women with endometriosis suffer from severe menstrual cramps (dysmenorrhea) with dull, aching pain in the pelvis, lower abdomen, and back. Endometriosis develops when endometrial cells from the lining of the uterus migrate to locations outside the uterus and implant themselves on the ovaries, intestines, and bladder. As the patient gets older, these misplaced cells grow, causing increasing pain.

There are no specific laboratory tests to diagnose endometriosis. The only way to diagnose endometriosis is to have a laparoscopy procedure in which the doctor looks into the abdomen using a fiberoptic instrument known as a laparoscope. The extent of the condition can be assessed and, if necessary, laser therapy can remove the large masses.

Poly-MVA offers a remarkably effective alternative treatment for endo-metriosis. By enhancing the function of the liver, Poly-MVA helps move blood out of the pelvis via the portal vein, and the endometriosis cells appear to implode and disappear. Although research is still needed to elucidate the exact mechanism of Poly-MVA in the treatment of endometriosis, it is clear that many women suffering from this debilitating condition can be helped by treatment with Poly-MVA.

POLY-MVA FOR PETS

The cancer epidemic has struck our animal companions, too. It appears that Poly-MVA can help and support them, as well. Veterinarians across the country are finding that Poly-MVA has remarkable cancer-suppressing and, in many cases, reversing effects in animals. Ask your veterinarian about Poly-MVA if you think your pet can benefit from it.

POLY-MVA AS PART OF A DAILY NUTRITIONAL REGIMEN

Those who use Poly-MVA as a nutritional supplement or as a treatment for cancer report that they feel more energetic almost immediately. This compound reenergizes cells, particularly those under stress. It is an ideal oral antioxidant that strengthens immune response and increases energy. Poly-

MVA helps the body to perform at optimal levels by "supercharging" the cells and supplying nutrients that can easily be assimilated. As a preventive agent, it helps to avoid the age-related breakdown mainly associated with free-radical damage to cellular structure and function, and, in the process, it decreases vulnerability to disease.

DOSAGE RECOMMENDATIONS

If you wish to take Poly-MVA for health maintenance and cancer prevention, take $\frac{1}{4}$ to 1 teaspoon per day as part of your regular daily regimen. For best absorption, it should be taken thirty minutes prior to eating or taking other supplements.

If you are fighting early-stage cancer, start with a loading dose of 8 teaspoons a day, divided into 2 teaspoons four times daily for at least two months. Then reduce your dosage to 2 teaspoons twice daily (for a total of 4 teaspoons per day), gradually reducing further to 1 to 2 teaspoons daily to maintain remission. If your cancer is more advanced, you may require the loading dose for a longer period. Enlist the guidance of your healthcare team to decide how long to take the higher dosage. Although some patients see quick changes in their medical condition, others need to take Poly-MVA for a minimum of two to four months before major changes are documented. If you don't notice an immediate difference, don't be concerned. On average, it takes four weeks before results are seen and felt. You may also consider consulting with your physician regarding the possibility of using intravenous Poly-MVA. Intravenous Poly-MVA given prior to oxidative therapies such as ozone therapy and hydrogen peroxide therapy is a very powerful method to jump-start the body to improve bioenergetic function.

When taking Poly-MVA for cancer, keep in mind that cancer cell "die-off" can cause temporary increases in cancer marker tests, such as the AMAS test, and that Poly-MVA may act as a paramagnetic contrast agent, which means that it can cause changes in MRI scans that can be mistaken for cancerous growths.

For maximum benefit, Poly-MVA users can refer to the Poly-MVA website or call AMARC Enterprises, the sole distributor of Poly-MVA, for specific instructions (see the Resources section). You may be able to locate a practitioner in your area who can guide you in an alternative program that includes Poly-MVA; review the list of providers on the Poly-MVA website.

FURTHER RECOMMENDATIONS

Based on existing research, taking high doses of other antioxidants is not recommended while taking Poly-MVA. However, if antioxidant therapy is deemed appropriate, Poly-MVA and the antioxidant(s) should be taken on an alternating schedule with several hours between therapies. For example, if you are taking vitamin C in doses of 3,000–5,000 milligrams per day, wait six hours after taking the vitamin C before taking Poly-MVA.

The use of nicotine products or steroid drugs will diminish the effectiveness of Poly-MVA. Smoking is obviously not a good idea for people who are fighting cancer, but high-dose steroids are sometimes used in cancer therapy. Only decrease steroid dosage with close physician supervision.

Conclusion

This book has introduced you to the origin and potential uses of the unique and remarkable compound Poly-MVA and other palladium lipoic complexes (LAPds). As time goes on, new research will undoubtedly reveal how beneficial Poly-MVA can be—not only in the treatment of cancer but also for psoriasis and other autoimmune disorders, for the prevention of brain damage caused by stroke, and for the promotion of optimal health, energy, and longevity.

LAPd compounds were specifically designed to support healthy cells with the goal of selectively destroying abnormal cells without harming non-cancerous cells. The manner in which Poly-MVA does so has yet to be completely explained, but the research and the success stories from cancer patients are compelling enough—and the substances nontoxic enough—to merit its use by anyone who wishes to reverse or prevent cancer.

Although a regimen of Poly-MVA can be expensive, the potential benefits far exceed the cost. Palladium at times has been more expensive than gold. At present, none of the palladium lipoic complexes are covered by health insurance. But the evidence in its favor is strong, and it is the hope of everyone involved in offering this product that those who need it will find a way to get it for themselves or their loved ones.

Poly-MVA is currently only available from AMARC (see Resources), but as more research is completed, Poly-MVA and other palladium lipoic complexes will likely become more widely available.

Resources

For information about how to order Poly-MVA or to find a physician who will guide you in its use, visit the Poly-MVA Survivors' Website at www.facr.net and search under keyword "POLYMVA," or call AMARC Enterprises, the sole distributor of Poly-MVA. Other helpful contact information is included below. Contact information is subject to change.

AMARC Enterprises, Inc.

2278-J Sweetwater Springs Blvd.,
  #309
Spring Valley, CA 91977
Phone: (619) 713-0430
E-mail: info@polymva.com
www.polymva.com
Sole distributor of Poly-MVA.

Foundation for Advancement of Cancer Research

539 Telegraph Canyon Road
Chula Vista, CA 91910
Phone: (866) 522-6237

Garnett McKeen Laboratory, Inc.

187 West Main Street
East Islip, NY 11730
Phone: (631) 218-3400
E-mail: newcode@aol.com
www.electrogenetics.com

Hope 4 Cancer Institute

482 W. San Ysidro Blvd., #1589
San Ysidro, CA 92173
Patient Response Line:
  (800) 670-9124
www.hope4cancer.com
An organization that can provide information and advice about Poly-MVA and other alternative cancer treatments.

Chip White

Association for Wholintegral
  Medicine, Inc.
Phone: (510) 843-1559
E-mail: chip@corp.net
Chip is a researcher with extensive knowledge of and experience with Poly-MVA and other alternative approaches to disease.

References

American Cancer Society. 2002. Prevention and early detection. Common questions about diet and cancer. http://www2.cancer.org (retrieved January 6, 2003; site now discontinued).

Antonawich, F. J., S. M. Fiore, and J. N. Davis. 1998. The effects of a lipoic acid/palladium complex on hippocampal progenitor cells. Abstract #857.10, 24:2161. Society for Neuroscience Meeting, Los Angeles, CA.

Bohm, D. On the Intuitive Understanding of Nonlocality as Implied by Quantum Theory. *Foundation of Physics,* vol. 5, 1975, pp. 96, 102.

Dossey, L. *Space, Time, and Medicine.* New York: Random House, 1982, p. 146.

Foundation for the Advancement in Cancer Research. June 21, 2003. White Paper. *Palladium Lipoic Complexes: An Overview of Function and Clinical Applications to Cancer Treatment.*

Garnett, Merrill. Synthetic DNA reductase. *Journal of Bioinorganic Chemistry* 1995; 59(2–3): 231.

———. November 26, 1993. Palladium complexes and methods for using same in the treatment of tumors or psoriasis. U.S. Patent 5,463,093, Oct. 31, 1995. U.S. Patent 5,463,093, filed Nov. 26, 1993, issued Oct. 31, 1995.

———. 2001. The communication between cells is key to understanding malignant change. International Symposium on Applications of Enzymes in Chemistry.

———. 2002. *Developmental electronic circuits in cancer: Research and treatment.* Garnett McKeen Medical Science Series, vol. 1, no. 2. (Islip, New York).

———. 2001. *Electrogenetics: Biological liquid crystal theory.* Garnett McKeen Medical Science Series, No. 1. New York: First Pulse Projects.

———. 2001. *First pulse: A personal journey in cancer research.* 2nd ed. New York: First Pulse Projects.

Garnett, Merrill, John L. Remo, and C. V. Krishnan. 2002. Developmental electronic pathways and carcinogenesis. Paper presented at the Sixth International Conference of Bioenergetic Medicine.

Garnett, Wade, and Merrill Garnett. 1996. Charge relay from molybdate oxyradicals to palladium-lipoic complex to DNA. Paper presented at the Conference on Oxygen Metabolites in Nonheme Metabollichemistry, June 23, 1996, Univ. of Minnesota.

Haskin, Charlene. A review of ribonucleotide reductase and the related group of enzymes. Unpublished paper.

Manning, Clark, and Vanrenen, Louis. *Bioenergetic Medicine East and West: Acupuncture and Homeopathy.* Berkeley, CA: North Atlantic Books, 1988, p. 24.

Ou, P., H. J. Tritschler, and S. P. Wolff. Thioctic (lipoic) acid: A therapeutic metal-chelating antioxidant? *Biochem Pharmacol* 1995 Jun 29;50(1):123–6.

Sanchez, Al, Sr. 2003. *Overcome cancer.* Chula Vista, CA: AMARC.

Walker, Morton. Cancer remission rates increase from use of the safe and effective lipoic acid palladium complex Poly-MVA. *The Townsend Letter for Doctors & Patients* Feb/Mar 2003.

White, Chip. A brief report on palladium lipoic acid reductase in the treatment of cancer. Unpublished paper.

Index

About the Authors

Robert D. Milne, M.D., graduated from the University of Southern California and the University of Missouri-Columbia School of Medicine. Board certified in family medicine, Dr. Milne has been practicing complementary medicine for over twenty years. He is a contributing author of *Alternative Medicine: The Definitive Guide* (1993) and co-author of the *Definitive Guide to Headaches* (1997). He is a frequent lecturer and practices integrative medicine in Las Vegas, Nevada.

Melissa Block, M.Ed., is a health journalist and author who lives in Southern California. She has authored and contributed to dozens of books, articles, and websites on alternative medicine, nutrition, and fitness topics. She holds a graduate degree in exercise physiology from the University of Virginia.

Printed in the USA
CPSIA information can be obtained
at www.ICGtesting.com
JSHW012010140824
68134JS00004B/103